THE ART OF FATHERHOOD: MASTERING THE BALANCING ACT

MOSES SUNDAY

TABLE OF CONTENT

INTRODUCTION

"The Art of Fatherhood: Mastering the Balancing Act" is an exploration of the intricate and rewarding journey that is modern fatherhood. In a world where the roles of dads are evolving rapidly, this book serves as a guiding light for those who aspire to not only be great fathers but also find harmony between the many facets of life.

In the pages that follow, we delve deep into the heart of fatherhood, navigating the uncharted waters of parenting while managing the myriad demands of career, relationships, and personal growth. With a blend of heartfelt anecdotes, practical advice, and expert insights, this book offers a roadmap for dads seeking to strike that delicate balance.

You'll discover how to nurture your children's development, from teaching important life lessons to creating cherished family memories. We explore the challenges of being a dadpreneur, the joys of quality

Time, and the vital importance of self-care to prevent burnout.

"The Art of Fatherhood" is not just a book; it's a companion for the modern dad, providing inspiration and guidance on how to master the intricate dance of parenthood. Join us on this transformative journey, where you'll find the tools and wisdom to craft a legacy of love, guidance, and laughter for your children while mastering the balancing act of fatherhood.

CHAPTER ONE

The New Dad's Dilemma: Juggling Diapers and Dreams

In the quiet hours of a sleepless night, as I cradled my newborn daughter in my arms, I couldn't help but feel a sense of awe and responsibility wash over me. Her tiny fingers wrapped around mine, and her eyes, filled with curiosity, locked onto my own. It was at that moment, the moment I became a father, that the realization of the monumental balancing act ahead hit me like a ton of bricks.

Becoming a father is a journey that many of us embark on with a mixture of excitement and trepidation. The arrival of a new life in the family is a miraculous event, but it also marks the beginning of a lifelong challenge – the challenge of mastering the delicate art of fatherhood.

This chapter delves into the heart of the "New Dad's Dilemma," a dilemma that resonates with countless fathers around the world. It's a dilemma that involves juggling the responsibilities of caring for a newborn while still nurturing our dreams and ambitions. It's a dance on a tightrope, where one misstep can have far-reaching consequences.

The Arrival of a New World

The birth of a child is an event that transforms a man's world. Suddenly, the routines, priorities, and aspirations that once seemed so clear become tangled in a web of uncertainty. The immediate needs of a baby, from midnight feedings to endless diaper changes, demand your full attention. And yet, as a new dad, you're not just responsible for these immediate needs; you're also the architect of your child's future.

In those early days, I found myself wrestling with a barrage of questions. How could I balance the demands of my career with the responsibilities of fatherhood? Could I continue to pursue my dreams and passions while being the best dad I could be? The answers were not immediately clear, and the weight of these questions was enough to keep any new parent up at night.

The Evolution of Fatherhood

As I embarked on this journey, I couldn't help but reflect on how fatherhood had evolved over the years. Gone were the days when a father's role was limited to being the breadwinner, returning home after a long day at work, and offering a few moments of paternal authority. Modern fatherhood was a dynamic, ever-changing role that demanded not just financial support but emotional presence, active engagement, and shared responsibilities in raising a child.

This shift in the concept of fatherhood was both a blessing and a challenge. While it opened up new opportunities for fathers to connect with their children on a deeper level, it also meant navigating uncharted territory. We were the pioneers of this new era of fatherhood, and we needed to find our way through the wilderness of parenting.

The Balancing Act Begins

To master the art of fatherhood, one must first embrace the balancing act it entails. The first step in this delicate dance is recognizing that the scales are not static; they will tip and sway, requiring constant adjustments. It's not about achieving a perfect equilibrium but rather learning to adapt and thrive amid the constant movement.

The balancing act involves three key elements: family, career, and personal growth. Each of these elements exerts its gravitational pull, and as a new dad, you'll often find yourself pulled in multiple directions simultaneously.

Family: Your family is your foundation, and as a father, your primary responsibility is to ensure the well-being and happiness of your spouse and children. This entails being present for the daily rituals of parenting, from changing diapers to bedtime stories and creating a nurturing environment where your children can flourish.

Career: For many fathers, career aspirations are deeply ingrained, and the desire to provide for your family financially is a powerful motivator. Balancing a thriving career with the demands of fatherhood requires careful planning and time management, as well as the ability to adapt to changing circumstances in the workplace.

Personal Growth: It's easy to forget about your dreams and aspirations when faced with the demands of parenthood, but personal growth is an essential part of the equation. As a father, you must continue to pursue your passions, hobbies, and self-improvement, not just for your fulfillment but also as a model for your children.

The New Dad's Toolbox

To navigate this complex terrain, you'll need a well-equipped toolbox. This toolbox is not filled with physical tools but rather with a set of principles and strategies that will serve as your guideposts on the journey of fatherhood.

1. Prioritization: At the core of the balancing act is the skill of prioritization. You must discern what truly matters most in each moment and make decisions accordingly. Sometimes, this means putting work on hold to comfort a crying baby and other times, it means carving out dedicated time for your pursuits.

2. Communication: Open and honest communication with your partner is necessary. Your spouse is your partner in this grand adventure, and together, you can navigate the challenges and joys of parenthood. Discuss your Expectations, fears, and aspirations, and work together to find common ground.

3. Support Network: No man is an island, and no father can go it alone. Building a support network of friends, family, and fellow fathers can provide invaluable guidance and a sense of community. Sharing experiences and advice can help you feel less isolated and more empowered as a father.

4. Flexibility: The ability to adapt and be flexible is a key skill for any new dad. Plans may change, unexpected challenges may arise, and the best-laid schemes may go awry. Embrace flexibility and learn to go with the flow, knowing that sometimes, the most memorable moments come from the unexpected.

5. Self-Care: Perhaps the most overlooked tool in the new dad's toolbox is self-care. Taking care of your physical and mental well-being is not a selfish act but a necessary one. When you are at your best, you can be the best father, partner, and individual.

Closing Thoughts

As I gazed down at my daughter on that sleepless night, I realized that the balancing act of fatherhood was not a burden but a privilege. It was an opportunity to shape a new life, to witness the growth and development of a tiny human being, and to be a source of love and guidance.

In the pages that follow, we will delve deeper into the intricacies of this balancing act. We will explore the challenges and triumphs of being a modern father, how we can foster strong family bonds, and the strategies for pursuing our dreams while nurturing our children.

This is the journey of the new dad, and it is a journey filled with both joy and complexity. As we embark on this adventure together, remember that you are not alone. Countless fathers have walked this path before, and countless more will follow. By sharing our experiences and wisdom, we can all strive to master the art of fatherhood and find that elusive balance between diapers and dream.

CHAPTER TWO

Becoming a Dadpreneur: Navigating Fatherhood and Career

In the modern world, the traditional lines that once separated work and family life have blurred. Nowhere is this more evident than in the lives of fathers who seek to excel both as dads and as entrepreneurs or professionals. This chapter delves into the intricate dance of becoming a "Dadpreneur," a term coined to describe those fathers who are navigating the challenging terrain of balancing fatherhood and a career they're passionate about.

The Dadpreneur Dilemma

The Dadpreneur's journey begins with a unique set of challenges. Unlike traditional roles where the boundaries between work and family are more defined, the Dadpreneur often finds himself in uncharted territory. The desire to build a successful career or business is strong, but so is the commitment to being an engaged and present father.

The Passion for Work

For many Dadpreneurs, the drive to excel in their careers or entrepreneurial ventures is a deeply ingrained passion. It's a fire that fuels their ambitions and propels them to pursue their dreams. This passion is what motivates them to take risks, overcome obstacles, and work tirelessly to achieve their goals.

The Love for Family

Simultaneously, the love and dedication these fathers feel toward their families are equally profound. The moments spent with their children are priceless, and they are committed to being there for the milestones, big and small, that shape their children's lives. The joy of being a father is a source of inspiration that drives them to create a better future for their families.

The Art of Integration

Navigating the Dadpreneur dilemma is an art, and it begins with integration. Instead of trying to compartmentalize work and family life, the Dadpreneur seeks to integrate the two in a way that allows them to coexist harmoniously. Here are some procedures to master this art:

1.   **Define Your Values:** The foundation of successful integration lies in understanding your values. What truly matters to you? What are your non-negotiable when it comes to both your career and your family? By defining your values, you can make informed decisions that align with your priorities.

2. **Set Clear Boundaries:** Boundaries are your allies in maintaining balance. Clearly define when you are "at work" and when you are "at home." Communicate these boundaries to your family and colleagues to ensure everyone understands your availability and expectations.

3. **Prioritize Tasks**: In both your career and family life, not all tasks are created equal. Prioritize your tasks based on significance and urgency. By focusing on high-priority tasks first, you can allocate more time to the things that matter most.

4. **Embrace Flexibility:** Life is unpredictable, and the ability to adapt and be flexible is essential. There will be

days when work demands more of your time and others when your family needs your attention. Embrace the ebb and flow of these demands without guilt.

5. Leverage Technology: In today's digital age, technology can be a valuable ally. Use tools and apps to streamline your work processes and communication, allowing you to be more efficient and free up time for your family.

6. Delegate and Seek Support: You don't have to do it all alone. Delegate tasks at work when possible and enlist the support of your partner or other family members in household and childcare responsibilities. A support system is invaluable.

7. Quality over Quantity: It's not about the quantity of time you spend with your family; it's about the quality of those moments. Be fully present during family time, put away distractions, and make the most of the time you have together.

Success Stories: Real-Life Dadpreneurs

To illustrate the concept of the Dadpreneur and the art of integration, let's look at a few real-life success stories:

1. Elon Musk

Elon Musk, the visionary behind SpaceX and Tesla, is not only a tech mogul but also a dedicated father to several children. Despite the demands of running multiple companies, Musk is known for making an effort to spend quality time with his kids, showing that even the busiest of Dadpreneurs can find balance.

2. Richard Branson

The charismatic founder of the Virgin Group, Richard Branson, has also embraced the role of Dadpreneur. He's managed to build an empire while maintaining a strong presence in the lives of his children, often involving them in his adventures and charitable work.

3. Mark Zuckerberg

Mark Zuckerberg, the co-founder of Facebook (now Meta Platforms, Inc.), is another example of a Dadpreneur who has successfully juggled Entrepreneurship and fatherhood. He's known for his dedication to both his company and his family, setting a positive example for fathers in the tech industry.

While these success stories are inspiring, it's essential to acknowledge that the path of the Dadpreneur is not without its challenges. There will be moments of exhaustion, tough decisions, and inevitable sacrifices. However, the rewards are immeasurable.

1. Fulfillment: The Dadpreneur experiences a unique sense of fulfillment that comes from not only pursuing their passions but also being present for their children's milestones. The satisfaction of watching your child take their first steps can be as exhilarating as closing a business deal.

2. Role Model: Dadpreneurs have the opportunity to be powerful role models for their children. They teach their kids the value of hard work, determination, and resilience by example. Children see firsthand what it means to chase dreams and never give up.

3. Legacy: By integrating their career aspirations with their commitment to family, Dadpreneurs are often on the path to leaving a meaningful legacy. They create businesses or achieve professional success that can benefit their children and future generations.

The journey of the Dadpreneur is a testament to the art of integration. It is a testament to the belief that, with careful planning, dedication, and a deep understanding of one's values, it is possible to excel in both the worlds of work and family.

As you embark on your own Dadpreneur journey, remember that there is no one-size-fits-all approach. Your path will be unique, and shaped by your values, circumstances, and aspirations. Embrace the challenges and rewards of this intricate dance, and know that the journey itself is a remarkable achievement. Mastering the art of being a Dadpreneur is not about achieving a perfect balance but about finding harmony between the two worlds you hold dear.

CHAPTER 3

Super Dad or Burnout: The Power of Self-Care

In the pursuit of being a super dad, many fathers often find themselves on the brink of burnout. The desire to provide, protect, and be present for their families drives them to give their all, but it can also lead to neglecting a critical aspect of their well-being – self-care. In this chapter, we explore the delicate balance between being a super dad and avoiding the pitfalls of burnout by harnessing the transformative power of self-care.

The Super Dad Myth

The Super Dad is a pervasive archetype in our society. He's strong, selfless, tireless, and always there for his family. He can leap tall buildings in a single bound, or at least it seems that way when we see fathers tirelessly juggling work, family, and countless responsibilities. While the intentions behind this image are admirable, the reality is often far more complex.

The Burnout Trap

When the pursuit of being a super dad comes at the expense of self-care, burnout becomes a looming threat. Burnout isn't just physical exhaustion; it's emotional and mental fatigue that can have profound consequences on a father's well-being, family life, and overall happiness.

Signs of Burnout

Recognizing the signs of burnout is crucial for any father. Here are some common indicators:

1. Chronic Fatigue: Feeling constantly drained, both physically and emotionally.

2. Increased Irritability: Becoming easily frustrated or irritable, even over minor issues.

3. Neglecting Self-Care: Failing to prioritize your well-being and neglecting hobbies or activities you once enjoyed.

4. Reduced Patience: Having less patience with your children or partner.

5. Loss of Interest: Losing interest in things that used to bring you joy.

6. Cynicism: Developing a negative or cynical outlook on life.

7. Physical Symptoms: Experiencing physical symptoms like headaches, digestive issues, or muscle tension.

If any of these sound familiar, it's essential to take them seriously. Burnout not only affects you but also has a ripple effect on your family.

The Power of Self-Care

Self-care isn't selfish; it's an act of self-preservation and, ultimately, an act of love toward your family. It's about recognizing that to be the best dad, partner, and person you can be, you need to take care of yourself first. Self-care isn't just an indulgence; it's a necessity for maintaining your physical and mental health.

Self-care encompasses a wide range of activities and practices that promote well-being. Here are some key categories of self-care:

1. Physical Self-Care: Physical self-care involves activities that enhance your physical health and vitality. This includes regular exercise, maintaining a balanced diet, getting enough sleep, and staying hydrated. Taking care of your body lays the foundation for a healthy and energized life.

2. Emotional Self-Care: Emotional self-care focuses on your emotional wellbeing. It involves recognizing and expressing your feelings, seeking support from friends or a therapist when needed, and engaging in activities that bring you joy and relaxation. Emotional self-care allows you to better manage stress and maintain healthy relationships.

3. Mental Self-Care: Mental self-care involves nurturing your cognitive wellbeing. This includes practicing mindfulness or meditation, reading, engaging in creative hobbies, and seeking intellectual stimulation. Keeping your mind sharp and engaged is essential for mental resilience.

4. Social Self-Care: Social self-care revolves around maintaining healthy relationships and connections. Spending quality time with loved ones, nurturing friendships, and seeking social support are crucial aspects of social self-care. Strong social connections provide emotional support and a sense of belonging.

5. Spiritual Self-Care: Spiritual self-care isn't necessarily religious; it's about finding meaning and purpose in life. This can involve practices like meditation, prayer, spending time in nature, or engaging in activities that align with your values. Spiritual self-care nourishes your inner self and fosters a sense of purpose.

Self-Care Strategies for Super Dads

Integrating self-care into your daily life demands intention and commitment. Here are some strategies to help you strike the right balance:

1. Prioritize Self-Care: Acknowledge that self-care is not a luxury but a necessity. Make it a priority in your daily routine, just like any other responsibility.

2. Schedule It: Set aside dedicated time for self-care activities. Block it off in your calendar to ensure it doesn't get pushed aside by other demands.

3. Communicate Your Needs: Don't hesitate to communicate your need for self-care to your partner and children. Let them know that taking care of yourself ultimately benefits the whole family.

4. Learn to Say No: it's okay to say no when you're feeling overwhelmed or stretched too thin. Setting boundaries is a vital part of self-care.

5. Seek Support: Consider joining a support group for fathers or seeking professional help if you're experiencing burnout or emotional distress. Periodically, talking to someone who understands can make a world of difference.

6. Small Steps Count: You don't need to overhaul your life to practice self-care. Little, consistent steps can have a significant impact. Whether it's taking a short walk, reading a book for 15 minutes, or practicing deep breathing exercises, these small moments of self-care add up.

Tom, a devoted father of two young children, found himself teetering on the edge of burnout. His job demanded long hours, and he often felt like he had no time for himself. His patience with his kids was wearing thin, and he constantly felt exhausted.

Recognizing the signs of burnout, Tom decided to prioritize self-care. He started waking up 30 minutes earlier each day to meditate and do some light stretching exercises. This allowed him to start his day with a sense of calm and focus. He also communicated his need for occasional breaks to his partner and took short walks during lunch breaks at work.

Over time, these small changes had a profound impact. Tom's energy levels improved, his patience with his children increased, and he felt more content overall. By embracing self-care, Tom not only prevented burnout but also became a better Super Dad for his family.

Conclusion

Being a Super Dad doesn't mean sacrificing your wellbeing on the altar of parenthood. Taking care of yourself is an essential part of being a Super Dad. By prioritizing self-care, you not only safeguard your

Health and happiness but also become a better father, partner, and person. Remember that self-care is a continuous journey, and it's never too late to start. Your well-being matters, and it's a cornerstone of your ability to provide love, support, and guidance to your family. Embrace the transformative power of self-care, and you'll discover the true strength of being a Super Dad.

CHAPTER FOUR

From Playdates to Date Nights: Balancing Family and Romance

As a father, it's natural to place your family at the center of your world. The joys of parenting, the laughter of your children, and the satisfaction of being there for them are priceless. Yet, amidst the hustle and bustle of family life, it's essential not to forget another crucial aspect of your life – your romantic relationship with your partner. Balancing family and romance is an art, and in this chapter, we'll explore how to keep the flame of love alive while nurturing your family bonds.

The Family Romance Connection

Romance and family life aren't mutually exclusive; they are deeply intertwined. The love and connection you share with your partner are the foundation on which your family is built. Strong romantic bonds between parents provide stability and emotional support for children, helping them feel secure and loved.

The Challenges of Balancing Family and Romance

Balancing the demands of family life with the desire for romance can be challenging. The responsibilities of parenting, work, and household chores often leave little time or energy for intimate moments with your partner. However, addressing these challenges is crucial to maintaining a healthy and fulfilling relationship.

Recognizing the Importance of Romance

Before diving into practical strategies, it's essential to recognize why maintaining romance in your relationship matters:

1. Connection: Romance fosters a deeper emotional connection between partners, which can strengthen your overall relationship.

2. Role Modeling: When children witness their parents in a loving, affectionate relationship, it sets a positive example for their future relationships.

3. Stress Reduction: Romance can serve as a stress reliever, helping both partners cope with the demands of parenting and work.

4. Passion and Intimacy: Keeping the spark alive in your relationship can lead to a more passionate and intimate connection.

Now, let's explore strategies to help you balance family and romance:

2. Prioritize Your Relationship: Just as you prioritize your family's needs, prioritize your relationship. Make a conscious effort to allocate time, energy, and attention to your partner. Set aside dedicated moments for each other, even amid a hectic schedule.

2. Communicate Openly: Effective communication is the cornerstone of a healthy relationship. Discuss your desires, needs, and concerns with your partner openly and honestly. This includes discussing how you can create more romantic moments together.

3. Schedule Date Nights: Regular date nights are essential for keeping the romance alive. Set a recurring date night, whether it's weekly or monthly, where you can focus solely on each other. Plan activities you both enjoy, whether it's a cozy dinner at home, a movie night, or an evening stroll.

4. Make Small Gestures Count: Romance doesn't always require grand gestures. Small acts of affection and thoughtfulness, such as leaving sweet notes, sending text messages, or surprising your partner with their favorite treat, can go a long way in expressing your love.

5. Share Parenting Responsibilities: Balancing family and romance involves equitable distribution of parenting responsibilities. Share the tasks of childcare, household chores, and school commitments, so both partners have time to relax and recharge.

6. Create Couple Time at Home: While date nights are crucial, it's also essential to create a couple time at home. After the kids are in bed, reserve some quiet moments for conversation, cuddling, or watching a movie together. These moments can be just as intimate and special as going out.

7. Seek Support: Don't hesitate to seek support from friends, family, or a trusted babysitter. Having a reliable person to look after your children can allow you and your partner to enjoy some quality time together without worries.

8. Revisit Shared Interests: Rekindle your connection by revisiting the interests and activities you enjoyed as a couple before becoming parents. Whether it's a shared hobby, a favorite vacation spot, or a particular sport, reliving these experiences can reignite the romance.

Case Study: Sarah and Mike

Sarah and Mike, parents of two energetic boys, faced the typical challenges of balancing family and romance. Both had demanding jobs, and their sons' schedules were filled with school, sports, and playdates. As a result, their once-vibrant relationship started to lose its spark.

Recognizing the need for change, Sarah and Mike decided to implement some strategies to revive their romance. They scheduled a monthly date night and took turns planning special evenings. They also sought help from a trusted friend for occasional babysitting, which allowed them to enjoy more quality time together.

Additionally, they started sharing more household responsibilities, ensuring that neither partner felt overwhelmed by chores or childcare duties. These changes not only brought them closer but also made their family life more manageable.

Conclusion

Balancing family and romance is an ongoing journey, and it requires effort, commitment, and creativity. The goal is not to strive for perfection but to create a loving and harmonious environment where both your family and romantic relationship can thrive. Remember that your relationship with your partner is a precious asset that deserves attention and care. By nurturing your romantic connection, you're not only enriching your lives as a couple but also setting a positive example for your children, showing them the power of love, commitment, and balance. So, from playdates to date nights, embrace the challenge of maintaining a loving Family and a passionate romance – it's a journey well worth taking.

CHAPTER FIVE

Teaching Moments: The Art of Parenting with Purpose

Parenting is a journey filled with countless teaching moments. From the first time you hold your child in your arms to the day they leave the nest, you have the incredible opportunity to shape their character, values, and worldview. In this chapter, we explore the art of parenting with purpose, focusing on how to make the most of these teaching moments and guide your children toward a fulfilling and meaningful life.

Parenting with purpose is about being intentional in your approach to raising children. It means recognizing that your role as a parent goes beyond providing for their physical needs; it involves nurturing their emotional and moral development. When you parent with purpose, you actively shape the values and principles your children carry with them into adulthood.

Identifying Teaching Moments

Teaching moments are often disguised as everyday experiences. They can arise from the simplest interactions or the most challenging situations. The key is to be attuned to them and seize the opportunity to impart valuable lessons. Here's how to identify teaching moments:

1. Observation: Pay attention to your child's actions, questions, and reactions. Often, their curiosity or behavior can lead to meaningful discussions.

2. Reflect on Your Values: Think about the values and principles you want to instill in your children. This clarity will help you recognize teaching moments that align with your family's core beliefs.

3. Everyday Situations: Everyday activities such as mealtime, bedtime, and chores provide excellent teaching moments. These routines offer a consistent platform for sharing values and reinforcing positive behavior.

Teaching Moments in Action

Let's explore some common scenarios where parenting with purpose can make a significant impact:

1. Handling Conflict: When siblings squabble or children experience disagreements with friends, use these moments to teach conflict resolution skills. Encourage them to communicate their feelings, listen to others, and find mutually beneficial solutions.

2. Gratitude and Empathy: Teaching your children to be thankful and empathetic is a lifelong lesson. Encourage them to express gratitude for the little things and empathize with others' feelings and experiences.

3. Responsibility and Accountability: Chores and responsibilities at home are excellent opportunities to teach accountability. When your child completes a task, acknowledge their effort, and discuss the importance of fulfilling responsibilities.

4. Mistakes and Learning: Everyone makes mistakes, and these moments can be some of the most valuable teaching opportunities. Encourage your child to learn from their errors, emphasizing that failure is a part of growth.

5. Resilience and Perseverance: When your child faces challenges, teach them the importance of resilience and perseverance. Share stories of your life experiences and how you overcame obstacles. Let them know that setbacks are temporary and that they can overcome difficulties with determination.

6. Kindness and Generosity: Model kindness and generosity in your actions and words. Encourage your children to perform acts of kindness, whether it's helping a friend, donating to a charity, or simply showing empathy to those in need.

7. Values and Ethics: Engage in discussions about values and ethics, addressing topics like honesty, integrity, respect, and fairness. Share stories and examples that illustrate these principles.

Now that you've identified teaching moments, it's time to consider strategies for parenting with purpose:

1. Lead by Example: Children often learn by observing their parents. Model the values and behaviors you wish to infuse into them. Your actions speak louder than words.

2. Create a Safe Space: Encourage open and honest communication by creating a safe space for your children to express their thoughts and feelings without fear of judgment. Be a good listener and validate their feelings.

3. Ask Open-Ended Questions: Engage your children in conversations by asking open-ended questions. Instead of asking, "How was school today?" try, "Tell me about your day. What was the best part, and what was challenging?"

4. Storytelling: Share personal stories, anecdotes, or fables that convey important life lessons. Stories have a powerful way of teaching values and principles.

5. Encourage Critical Thinking: Challenge your children to think critically about various situations. Ask them how they would handle specific scenarios and discuss the potential consequences of their choices.

6. Set Clear Boundaries: While encouraging independence, it's important to set clear boundaries that align with your family's values. Boundaries provide a framework for ethical decision making.

7. Reinforce Positive Behavior: Celebrate and acknowledge moments when your children display positive behavior. Positive reinforcement encourages them to continue making ethical choices.

Case Study: The Anderson Family

The Anderson family consists of two parents, Sarah and David, and their two children, Emma and Liam. Sarah and David are committed to parenting with purpose and making the most of teaching moments.

One evening at the dinner table, Emma shared a story about a classmate who was being excluded by their group of friends. Sarah and David saw this as a teaching moment. They engaged the children in a discussion about kindness and empathy. They asked open-ended questions like, "How do you think that kid feels?" and "What can you do to be a friend to someone who feels left out?"

This conversation became a regular part of their dinner routine, and it reinforced the values of inclusivity and empathy in Emma and Liam. Over time, the children started inviting classmates who were on the fringes of social circles to join them for lunch or playdates, demonstrating the power of parenting with purpose in action.

Conclusion

Parenting with purpose is a journey that requires dedication, intentionality, and patience. It involves recognizing the teaching moments that arise in everyday life and seizing them as opportunities to instill values, ethics, and life lessons in your children. Remember that your role as a parent is not just to nurture their physical well-being but also to guide their moral and emotional development. By embracing these teaching moments, you empower your children to navigate the complexities of life with wisdom, empathy, and purpose, setting them on a path toward a fulfilling and meaningful future.

CHAPTER SIX

The Digital Dad: Managing Screens and Bonding Time

In today's digital age, screens have become an integral part of our lives, offering both opportunities and challenges, especially for fathers. The role of the "Digital Dad" involves navigating the digital landscape while ensuring that screens don't become barriers to meaningful family bonding. In this chapter, we'll explore how to manage screens effectively and find the right balance between technology and quality family time.

The Digital Age Dilemma

The proliferation of smartphones, tablets, and computers has transformed the way families interact and spend their time. While technology can offer educational and entertainment benefits, it also presents a set of challenges for parents. The

Digital Dad is tasked with managing screens and ensuring that they enhance, rather than hinder, family connections.

The Importance of Family Bonding

Family bonding is essential for children's emotional development and overall well-being. It provides a sense of security, belonging, and support that shapes their self-esteem and social skills. Quality family time also allows parents to impart values and life lessons to their children.

The Impact of Screens on Family Bonding

Excessive screen time can have adverse effects on family bonding. When screens dominate family life, they can lead to decreased communication, reduced physical activity, and a lack of meaningful interaction. Digital Dads must strike a balance that allows technology to coexist harmoniously with family time.

Managing Screens as a Digital Dad

Balancing screens and family bonding involves a combination of strategies and mindful choices. Here are some effective ways to manage screens as a Digital Dad:

1. Set Screen Time Limits: Establish clear screen time limits for both children and adults in the family. Create a schedule that designates specific times for screen use, such as after homework or chores are completed. Stick to these limits consistently.

2. Model Healthy Screen Habits: Children often mimic their parents' behavior. Set a positive example by practicing healthy screen habits yourself. Demonstrate that screens are tools for communication, learning, and entertainment, but they shouldn't dominate your life.

3. Designate Screen-Free Zones: Create screen-free zones in your home, such as the dining room and bedrooms. These areas should be reserved for family meals, conversations, and relaxation without the distraction of screens.

4. Engage in Digital Detox Days: Occasionally, plan digital detox days where the entire family disconnects from screens. Use this time to engage in outdoor activities, board games, or creative projects that promote quality bonding.

5. Prioritize Face-to-Face Conversations: Encourage face-to-face conversations with your children. Ask about their day, interests, and concerns. These conversations provide opportunities to connect on a deeper level and demonstrate that you value their thoughts and feelings.

6. Choose High-Quality Content: When screen time is allowed, prioritize high-quality content that is both educational and entertaining. There are plenty of apps, games, and shows that offer valuable learning experiences for children.

7. Screen Co-viewing: Whenever possible, engage in screen activities with your children. Co-viewing or co-playing allows you to bond over shared interests and opens up avenues for discussion and learning.

Case Study: The Johnson Family

The Johnson family consisted of two working parents, Mark and Lisa, and their two children, Ava and Ethan. Recognizing the challenges of managing screens, they implemented a screen time plan.

Mark and Lisa set screen time limits for Ava and Ethan, allowing them a certain amount of screen time each day after completing homework and chores. They also established a weekly family movie night, where they watched age-appropriate films together, followed by discussions about the movie's themes and lessons.

To model healthy screen habits, Mark and Lisa designated screen-free zones in their home, such as the dining room and bedrooms. During family meals, they encouraged open conversations without screens, reinforcing the importance of face-to-face interactions.

They also planned digital detox weekends once a month, during which screens were turned off, and the family engaged in outdoor activities, board games, and cooking together. These detox weekends became cherished moments of connection for the Johnson family.

The Benefits of Balancing Screens and Bonding Time

Balancing screens and family bonding offers numerous benefits for both children and parents:

1. Stronger Family Connections: Quality family time strengthens the emotional bonds between parents and children, fostering a sense of security and love.

2. Enhanced Communication: Limiting screen time encourages face-to-face communication, allowing parents and children to share experiences, thoughts, and feelings more openly.

3. Improved Emotional Well-being: Reducing screen time can lead to decreased stress and anxiety levels, promoting overall emotional wellbeing for both children and adults.

4. Enhanced Creativity: Engaging in screen-free activities stimulates creativity, problem-solving, and imaginative play, which are essential for children's development.

5. Opportunities for Learning: Balancing screens with other activities provides opportunities for learning through play, exploration, and hands-on experiences.

6. Positive Role Modeling: By managing screens effectively, Digital Dads can model healthy habits and behaviors that their children will carry with them into adulthood.

Conclusion

The Digital Dad faces the challenge of managing screens in a digital age while nurturing meaningful family bonds. By setting clear screen time limits, modeling healthy screen habits, designating screen free zones, and prioritizing face-to-face interactions, you can strike the right balance between technology and quality family time.

Remember that the goal isn't to eliminate screens but to use them purposefully and mindfully. By doing so, you can create a home environment where screens enhance family life rather than detract from it. The result will be stronger family connections, improved communication, and opportunities for your children to learn and grow in a healthy, balanced way. Balancing screens and bonding time is an ongoing journey that can lead to a happier, more connected family life in

CHAPTER SEVEN

The Coach, Chef, and Clown: Multitasking in Fatherhood.

Being a dad often feels like taking on multiple roles simultaneously. You're not just a parent; you're also a coach, chef, clown, and so much more. Multitasking in fatherhood is an art, and in this chapter, we'll explore the challenges and rewards of juggling these roles while striving to be the best father you can be.

The Multitasking Dad

From the moment you become a dad, you quickly realize that parenthood is a multifaceted journey. It's not just about providing for your children's basic needs; it's about being a source of support, guidance, and love. This involves wearing various hats and seamlessly transitioning between roles to meet the ever-changing demands of fatherhood.

The Coach

As a dad, you often find yourself in the role of a coach. Whether it's teaching your child how to ride a bike, throwing a baseball, or helping with homework, you become their primary source of guidance and encouragement. Coaching isn't just about skill building; it's about instilling confidence and a sense of accomplishment in your child.

The Chef

Dads frequently step into the kitchen as the chef of the family. Preparing meals that are not only nutritious but also delicious becomes a part of your routine. Cooking for your family is an opportunity to bond, create traditions, and share the joy of good food.

The Clown

Laughter is a universal language of love, and dads often find themselves playing the role of the family clown. You tell silly jokes, make funny faces, and engage in playful antics to bring smiles and laughter to your children's faces. Being the clown creates cherished memories and strengthens your connection.

The Disciplinarian

While dads love to have fun, they're also responsible for setting boundaries and enforcing rules. The disciplinarian role is about teaching your children values, responsibility, and consequences for their actions. It's a tough role but essential for their growth and development.

The Listener

Listening plays a vital role in Fatherhood. Your children come to you with their worries, dreams, and questions. Being an attentive and empathetic listener allows you to provide emotional support and guidance when they need it most.

The Provider

As the provider, you work hard to ensure your family's financial stability. This role involves making financial decisions, planning for the future, and creating a secure environment for your children to thrive.

The Multitasking Challenge

Balancing these roles is undoubtedly a challenge. There are moments when you're simultaneously coaching your child in a sport, managing a simmering pot on the stove, and cracking jokes to keep everyone entertained. The multitasking dad often faces exhaustion and time constraints, which can lead to feelings of overwhelm.

While multitasking in dad-hood is demanding, there are strategies to help you navigate these various roles effectively and with confidence:

1. Prioritize Quality over Quantity: It's not about how many roles you can play at once, but how well you can fulfill them. Prioritize quality interactions with your children, even if they are brief.

2. Create a Routine: Establishing a daily routine can help you allocate time for each role. Having a structured schedule ensures that you can meet your children's needs without feeling rushed or overwhelmed.

3. Involve Your Children: Engage your children in some of your roles. Encourage them to help with cooking, be your assistant coach, or participate in family discussions. Involving them fosters a sense of responsibility and teamwork.

4. Embrace Flexibility: Flexibility is key to successful multitasking. Be prepared to adapt when things don't go as planned. Life is full of surprises, and being a dad means rolling with the punches.

5. Practice Self-Care: Don't forget to take care of yourself. Balancing multiple roles can be exhausting, so ensure you get enough rest, exercise, and moments of relaxation to recharge.

6. Seek Support: Don't be afraid to ask for help from your spouse, family members, or friends. Parenting is a team effort, and having a support system can make multitasking more manageable.

Case Study: The Williams Family

The Williams family consisted of Mark, a dedicated dad, his wife Sarah, and their three children. Mark was a coach, chef, and clown rolled into one. He juggled a demanding job, coaching his son's soccer team, preparing family meals, and making time for laughter.

To manage his roles effectively, Mark created a weekly schedule that allocated specific times for coaching, cooking, and playtime with his kids. He involved his children in meal preparation, turning cooking into a fun and educational activity. Mark also encouraged his kids to share their thoughts and feelings, fostering open communication.

Despite the challenges, Mark's dedication to balancing his roles paid off. His children thrived in their various activities, felt supported and loved, and enjoyed the sense of humor that permeated their home.

The Rewards of Multitasking in Fatherhood

While multitasking in dad-hood can be demanding, it comes with significant rewards:

1. Stronger Family Bonds: Balancing various roles allows you to connect with your children on multiple levels, strengthening your family bonds.

2. Personal Growth: Juggling multiple roles challenges you to grow personally. You develop patience, adaptability, and resilience, which can benefit you in all aspects of life.

3. Lifelong Memories: Your children will carry with them cherished memories of your coaching, cooking, and clowning. These moments become part of their narratives.

4. Role Model: As a multitasking dad, you become a role model for your children, showing them the importance of dedication, responsibility, and love in all that you do.

Conclusion

Multitasking in Fatherhood is a multi-faceted journey that requires dedication, adaptability, and a sense of humor. Embrace your various roles as a coach, chef, clown, and more with the understanding that each role contributes to your children's growth and your family's well-being. By prioritizing quality interactions, creating routines, involving your children, and seeking support when needed, you can successfully navigate the challenges and rewards of being a multitasking dad. In doing so, you create a loving and dynamic family environment where your children feel cherished, supported, and inspired to be the best they can be.

CHAPTER EIGHT

Adventure Awaits: Creating Memorable Family Experiences

Family life is a tapestry woven from countless moments, and among the most precious are the ones filled with adventure and shared experiences. In this chapter, we'll explore the importance of creating memorable family adventures, from simple day trips to epic journeys, and how these experiences strengthen bonds, build lasting memories, and enrich the tapestry of your family's story.

The Value of Family Adventures

Family adventures are more than just vacations or outings; they're opportunities for bonding, learning, and growth. These shared experiences have profound and lasting effects on family dynamics and individual development.

Strengthening Bonds

When families embark on adventures together, they create lasting memories and shared stories that bind them closer. Whether it's conquering a hiking trail, exploring a new city, or simply spending a day at the beach, these shared experiences become the fabric of your family's unique narrative.

Building Memories

Family adventures create memories that children carry with them into adulthood. These memories become a source of comfort, nostalgia, and inspiration throughout their lives. Recollections of a camping trip, a visit to a historical site, or a family road trip can bring warmth and joy even decades later.

Enriching Learning

Adventure is a powerful teacher. It exposes family members to new cultures, environments, and ideas. It broadens horizons, deepens understanding, and instills a sense of curiosity and wonder. Whether exploring a museum, visiting a wildlife sanctuary, or navigating a bustling marketplace, family adventures are rich with educational opportunities.

Nurturing Resilience

Challenges and unexpected situations are inevitable on adventures. These moments provide opportunities for family members to work together, solve problems, and develop resilience. Facing and overcoming obstacles as a team strengthens family bonds and builds confidence.

Creating Traditions

Family adventures often become cherished traditions. They are events that family members eagerly anticipate and look forward to year after year. Whether it's an annual camping trip, a holiday getaway, or a summer road trip, these traditions create a sense of continuity and connection.

Planning Memorable Family Adventures

Now that we've explored the value of family adventures, let's delve into the practical aspects of planning and experiencing them:

1. **Choose Age-Appropriate Adventures:** Consider the ages and interests of your family members when planning adventures. Opt for activities and destinations that are suitable for everyone. Be mindful of physical abilities, attention spans, and comfort levels.

2. Set Realistic Expectations: While adventure often involves stepping out of your comfort zone, it's essential to set realistic expectations. Plan activities that align with your family's interests and capabilities. Avoid over-scheduling or trying to fit too much into a single day.

3. Involve Everyone in Planning: Include your children in the planning process. Let them have a say in choosing destinations or workouts. Their involvement not only makes them feel valued but also adds an element of excitement as they look forward to the adventure.

4. Embrace Spontaneity: While planning is important, leave room for spontaneity. Some of the most memorable family adventures are born from unexpected detours or unplanned discoveries. Be open to exploring what comes your way.

5. Capture the Moments: Take plenty of photos and videos to capture the highlights of your family's adventures. These visual records will become treasured mementos that you can revisit and share with future generations.

6. Disconnect from Screens: While it's tempting to document every moment on social media, consider disconnecting from screens during your adventures. Engage fully in the experience, savoring the sights, sounds, and feelings of the moment.

7. Practice Safety: Safety should always be a priority on family adventures. Pack necessary supplies, follow safety guidelines, and be prepared for unexpected situations. Teaching your children about safety in various environments is an essential part of the adventure.

8. Reflect and Share: After each adventure, take time as a family to reflect on the experience. Share what you learned, your favorite moments, and any challenges you faced. This reflection process deepens the impact of the adventure and encourages open communication.

Case Study: The Garcia Family's National Park Expedition

The Garcia family, consisting of parents Luis and Maria and their two children, Sofia and Carlos, embarked on an unforgettable adventure to explore national parks. They planned a two-week road trip to visit several national parks, including Yosemite, Grand Canyon, and Yellowstone.

The trip required careful planning, as it involved long drives, camping, and hiking. Sofia and Carlos were involved in choosing the parks and activities they wanted to experience. They each had a journal to document their adventures, and the family agreed to disconnect from screens during most of the trip to immerse themselves fully in nature.

The journey was filled with awe-inspiring moments, from witnessing Old Faithful erupt at Yellowstone to hiking through the majestic landscapes of Yosemite. Along the way, the Garcia's learned about the importance of preserving natural environments, developed their outdoor skills, and deepened their appreciation for the beauty of the natural world.

Conclusion

Family adventures are the threads that weave the tapestry of your family's story. They create memories, strengthen bonds, and offer invaluable opportunities for growth and learning. Whether you're exploring distant lands or embarking on a simple weekend getaway, these adventures are the chapters that make your family's narrative vibrant

As a parent, you have the power to shape your children's perspectives and values through these shared experiences. The adventures you embark upon become the backdrop against which your family's unique story unfolds. So, embrace the spirit of adventure, plan memorable journeys, and savor every moment of discovery and connection with your loved ones. Adventure awaits, and it's an invitation to create a lifetime of cherished memories.

CHAPTER NINE

Raising Tomorrow's Leaders: Nurturing Character and Values

As a father, you play a pivotal role in shaping the future leaders of tomorrow. Beyond providing for their material needs, your influence extends into the realm of character and values. In this chapter, we explore the essential principles and strategies for nurturing character and instilling values in your children, setting them on a path to become responsible, compassionate, and ethical leaders.

The Foundation of Leadership

Leadership isn't merely about holding positions of authority; it's about guiding others with integrity, empathy, and a sense of purpose. True leaders inspire, empower, and make ethical decisions. As a father, you have the opportunity to lay the foundation for these qualities in your children.

1. Lead by Example: The most powerful way to instill values in your children is by embodying those values in your own life. Children learn through observation, so your actions, attitudes, and behaviors serve as a blueprint for their character development.

2. Teach Empathy: Empathy is a cornerstone of ethical leadership. Encourage your children to evaluate the feelings and standpoints of others. Engage in discussions about kindness, compassion, and the importance of treating everyone with respect.

3. Foster Responsibility: Responsibility is a fundamental aspect of character. Assign age-appropriate tasks and responsibilities to your children, such as chores, caring for pets, or managing their belongings. This teaches them accountability and the value of fulfilling commitments.

4. Encourage Critical Thinking: Critical thinking is essential for ethical decision-making. Engage your children in discussions that challenge them to think critically about ethical dilemmas and complex issues. Encourage them to ask questions and explore multiple perspectives.

5. Promote Integrity: Integrity is at the heart of ethical leadership. Teach your children the importance of honesty, truthfulness, and standing up for what is right, even when it's challenging. Discuss the consequences of dishonesty and the rewards of integrity.

6. Cultivate Resilience: Resilience is the ability to bounce back from setbacks and misfortune. Help your children develop resilience by teaching them to cope with challenges, learn from failures, and persevere in the face of obstacles.

7. Emphasize Teamwork: Leadership often involves working collaboratively with others. Encourage teamwork through group activities, sports, or volunteer opportunities. Teach your children the value of cooperation, communication, and compromise.

8. Cultivate a Growth Mindset: Foster a growth mindset in your children by emphasizing the importance of effort and learning from mistakes. Teach them that abilities can be developed through dedication and hard work, promoting a sense of self-improvement.

The Mitchell family consisted of parents, John and Lisa, and their two children, Mia and Ethan. John and Lisa were passionate about serving their community and instilling the value of service in their children.

The family regularly volunteered at a local food bank and participated in community cleanup events. Through these experiences, Mia and Ethan learned about the importance of giving back and helping those in need. John and Lisa also engaged their children in discussions about the impact of their actions on the community and the value of empathy.

As Mia and Ethan grew older, they took on more leadership roles within their volunteer activities, organizing food drives and charity events. These experiences not only taught them the importance of service but also developed their leadership skills, setting them on a path to become compassionate and responsible leaders in their own right.

Beyond specific strategies, nurturing character and values is an ongoing process woven into the fabric of everyday life. Here are some practical ways to infuse character development into your daily interactions with your children:

1. Family Meetings: Hold regular family meetings to discuss values, goals, and expectations. Encourage open dialogue and involve your children in decision-making processes.

2. Storytelling: Share stories and anecdotes that exemplify the values you want to instill. These stories can come from your own experiences, literature, history, or current events.

3. Reflection and Gratitude: Teach your children the practice of reflection and gratitude. Encourage them to express gratitude for the blessings in their lives and reflect on their actions and their impact on others.

4. Acts of Kindness: Model acts of kindness and encourage your children to perform random acts of kindness. These gestures can be as simple as helping a neighbor, donating to a charity, or volunteering as a family.

5. Mentorship: Provide opportunities for your children to learn from mentors or role models who embody the values you want to instill. This could be a family friend, teacher, coach, or community leader.

6. Community Involvement: Engage in community service or advocacy together as a family. Involvement in community issues can help your children develop a sense of social responsibility.

7. Encourage Independence: Allow your children to make age-appropriate decisions and face the consequences of their choices. Independence fosters a sense of responsibility and accountability.

8. Celebrate Achievements: Acknowledge and celebrate your children's achievements, both big and small. Recognize their efforts, persistence, and growth in character.

Conclusion

As a father, you have the extraordinary privilege and responsibility of nurturing character and values in your children, shaping them into tomorrow's leaders. Your guidance, example, and dedication to instilling empathy, responsibility, integrity, and resilience will have a profound impact on their lives and the lives of those they will lead.

Remember that character development is a lifelong journey, and it begins at home. Embrace your role as a mentor, teacher, and guide, and be mindful of the values you model in your daily life. By fostering these qualities, you empower your children to become ethical, compassionate, and responsible leaders who contribute positively to their communities and the world. In raising tomorrow's leaders, you leave a lasting legacy of character and values that will endure for generations to come.

CHAPTER TEN

Legacy Building: Leaving Your Mark on Your Children's Lives

As a father, you possess the unique opportunity to shape the legacy you leave behind in the hearts and minds of your children. Beyond material possessions, your true legacy is the impact you have on their character, values, and the way they navigate the world. In this chapter, we delve into the art of legacy building, exploring how you can create a lasting and meaningful imprint on your children's lives.

Defining Your Legacy

Before you can build a legacy, it's essential to clarify what you want it to encompass. Your legacy extends beyond your lifetime, so consider the long-lasting effects you hope to achieve. Some aspects to consider in defining your legacy include:

1. Values and Principles: What core values and principles do you want to instill in your children? Consider the moral and ethical beliefs that are important to you and that you want to pass on.

2. Life Lessons: Reflect on the life lessons and wisdom you've gained through your experiences. What insights do you want to share with your children to help them navigate their journeys?

3. Family Traditions and Stories: Family traditions and stories carry the essence of your family's history. What traditions do you want to preserve, and what stories do you want to pass down to future generations?

4. Giving Back and Service: Consider the legacy of service and giving back. How can you instill a sense of responsibility and compassion in your children, encouraging them to make a positive impact on their communities?

5. Personal Growth and Achievement: What personal achievements or goals do you hope your children will strive for? How can you inspire them to pursue their passions and reach their full potential?

Building a meaningful legacy requires intentionality and effort. Here are strategies to help you create a lasting impact on your children's lives:

1. Lead by Example: The most powerful way to shape your legacy is by living according to the values and principles you want to instill in your children. Model the behaviors and attitudes you hope they will emulate.

2. Open and Honest Communication: Foster open and honest communication with your children. Create an environment where they feel comfortable discussing their thoughts, feelings, and questions. Encourage them to share their philosophies and fears.

3. Storytelling and Shared Experiences: Share family stories and experiences that illustrate your values and the lessons you've learned. These stories become a part of your family's legacy and can inspire your children.

4. Document Your Wisdom: Consider creating a "legacy document" where you record your insights, life lessons, and personal philosophies. This document can serve as a source of guidance and inspiration for your children in the future.

5. Family Traditions: Establish and maintain family traditions that reflect your values and bring your family closer. These traditions can be as simple as weekly family dinners or more elaborate celebrations of holidays and milestones.

6. Encourage Independence: Empower your children to make their own choices and decisions. Encouraging independence and critical thinking allows them to grow and develop while still carrying your legacy with them.

7. Recognize Their Individuality: Acknowledge and celebrate your children's unique strengths, interests, and talents. Your legacy should support their individual growth and aspirations.

8. Encourage Generosity: Instill a sense of responsibility and generosity in your children by involving them in acts of kindness and community service. Show them the value of making a positive impact on the lives of others.

The Lewis family, consisting of parents Alex and Emily and their two children, Lily and Max, prioritized leaving a legacy of compassion. They volunteered regularly at a local homeless shelter, teaching their children the importance of helping those in need.

In addition to their volunteer work, the Lewis family established a tradition of "giving back" on each family member's birthday. Instead of receiving gifts, they chose a charitable cause to support as a family. This tradition instilled a sense of responsibility and generosity in Lily and Max, who grew up with a deep understanding of the impact they could have on the world.

As Lily and Max reached adulthood, they continued their family's legacy of compassion. They became advocates for social justice, supporting causes they were passionate about, and volunteering in their communities. The Lewis family's legacy of compassion lived on through the actions and values of their children.

The true essence of legacy building lies in passing down your values to your children. Here are ways to ensure that your values endure:

1. Consistency: Consistency is key in teaching values. Live out your values consistently, so your children witness their importance in action.

2. Reflection and Discussion: Engage in reflective discussions with your children about values, ethics, and the lessons they've learned from your experiences.

3. Encourage Critical Thinking: Encourage your children to think critically about their values and the values they want to uphold. Discuss various perspectives and help them make informed choices.

4. Celebrate Achievements: Celebrate moments when your children demonstrate the values you've instilled in them. Acknowledge and reward their efforts to reinforce the importance of these principles.

Legacy building is an ongoing journey, and as a father, you are a steward of the values and principles you hope to pass on to your children. Your legacy is not measured by the material possessions you leave behind but by the lasting impact you have on your children's character, values, and the positive contributions they make to the world.

By leading by example, fostering open communication, sharing stories and experiences, and encouraging independence and generosity, you can create a legacy that lives on through your children and their children, shaping the world for generations to come.

Your influence extends far beyond your lifetime, leaving a meaningful imprint on the hearts and minds of your family and the future leaders you are nurturing. Embrace the art of legacy building, and know that your values will endure as a guiding light for your children's journey through life.

www.ingramcontent.com/pod-product-compliance
Lightning Source LLC
Chambersburg PA
CBHW080728260726
48660CB00010B/3748